For Healing

by
Norvel Hayes

HARRISON HOUSE
Tulsa, Oklahoma

All Scripture quotations are taken from the *King James Version* of the Bible.

05 04   16 15

What To Do for Healing
ISBN 0-89274-216-X
Copyright © 1981 by Norvel Hayes
P.O. Box 1379
Cleveland, Tennessee 37311

Published by Harrison House, Inc.
P. O. Box 35035
Tulsa, Oklahoma 74153

What To Do For Healing

As I was preparing to minister on God's healing power one time, God gave me three passages of Scripture that show what the people in the Bible did to receive healing from Him. People today should do these same things.

The Lunatic Son

The first example is in Matthew, chapter 17:

When they were come to the multitude, there came to him a certain man, kneeling down to him (v. 14). The man evidently is coming to Jesus for some kind of help. What did he do when he came to Jesus? He knelt down.

The man said, *Lord, have mercy on my son: for he is a lunatic, and sore vexed: for ofttimes he falleth into the fire, and oft into the water. I brought him to thy disciples, and they could not cure him* (w. 15,16).

1

Jesus said, *O faithless and perverse generation, how long shall I be with you? how long shall I suffer you? Bring him hither to me* (v. 17).

The first words Jesus spoke when He heard that His disciples had not been able to cure the lunatic were: *O faithless.* Faithless means "no faith."

Jesus was talking about the disciples; but He told the father to bring his son to Him. Why? Because the father expressed his faith when he knelt down before Jesus and said, "Have mercy on my son." The moment he approached Jesus and spoke in faith, Jesus went to work on his behalf.

Jesus rebuked the devil; and he departed out of him: and the child was cured from that very hour (v.18). What did Jesus do? He rebuked the devil.

"Do you mean, Brother Norvel, that people in mental institutions have devils?" That's right. God doesn't make people sick or crazy.

All good things that come to you and your house come down from heaven. (James 1:17.) All bad things that come to the human race are from Satan—the god of darkness, the god of this world—and his workers, the demons. Jesus and His workers, the angels from heaven, are here to bless you and encourage you to believe the Bible.

The Bible says, *The child was cured from that very hour*. Can you imagine all the years of torment that child must have gone through? But he was completely normal in *that very hour*—in sixty minutes or less!

The Devil-Possessed Daughter

The second Scripture God gave me about an incident of healing is Matthew 15:21-28:

Jesus went thence, and departed into the coasts of Tyre and Sidon. And, behold, a woman of Canaan came out of the same coasts, and cried unto him, saying, Have mercy on me, O Lord, thou Son of David; my daughter is grievously vexed with a devil. But he answered her not a word...

Then came she and worshipped him, saying, Lord, help me. But he answered and said, It is not meet to take the children's bread, and to cast it to dogs. And she said, Truth, Lord: yet the dogs eat of the crumbs which fall from their masters' table.

Then Jesus answered and said unto her, O woman, great is thy faith: be it unto thee even as thou wilt. And her daughter was made whole from that very hour.

The disciples tried to send her away, but she worshipped Jesus, telling Him, "You can call me a dog if You want to. I'll even eat the crumbs that fall from Your table because You are my Master, Jesus, and I worship You."

The devil-possessed daughter who needed healing wasn't there in person—she was in another town—but the Spirit of God made her whole again in sixty minutes or less.

I want you to notice something: The healing didn't result until after the woman approached Jesus in reverence and asked Him in faith to help her.

The Leper

The first two Scripture passages God gave me about healing concerned children. This third one from Mark chapter 1, is for the individual:

And there came a leper to him, beseeching him, and kneeling down to him (v. 40). Again, we see that the person who came to Jesus for healing knelt down to Him and worshipped Him.

Today, cancer in certain stages is diagnosed by doctors in this country as incurable. In the days that Jesus walked the earth, leprosy was incurable.

This leper said to Jesus, *If thou wilt, thou canst make me clean* (v. 40). Some people think this statement expresses doubt. At the beginning, it sounds as though it does; but the last part is saying, "You *can* heal me, Jesus." This leper is expressing faith with his mouth.

And Jesus, moved with compassion, put forth his hand, and touched him, and saith unto him, I will; be thou clean. And as soon as he had spoken, immediately the leprosy departed from him, and he was cleansed (vv. 41,42).

They Worshipped and Received

In Matthew 17, the man knelt down before Jesus and said, "Jesus, have mercy on my son. He is a lunatic and is possessed with devils." When they brought the boy to Jesus, he was healed *from that very hour*.

In Matthew 15, the woman knelt down before Jesus and said, "You're my Master, Jesus. I worship You, Lord." Even though her devil-possessed daughter was in another town, she was made whole *from that very hour*.

In Mark 1, the leper knelt down to Jesus and said, *Thou canst make me clean*. When Jesus touched him, he was healed immediately.

In the first two instances, the parents wanted healing and deliverance for their children. In the third, a man wanted healing for himself.

In all three examples, the people sought God in the same way: They approached Jesus through worship by kneeling down before Him; and they expressed faith to Him through their words.

God responded in each case by healing them immediately.

Know That Jesus Heals

To receive healing, you must know, once and for all, that **Jesus heals people today.**

I'm not saying the devil won't attack you. He will. He will tell you: "You have been a Christian for so long. You know how much the Lord loves you. If He wanted to heal you, He would." That's not in the Scriptures. The Bible says God wants to heal everybody.

You also have to get it settled from the Bible that **healing is for you.** Jesus is no respecter of persons. (Acts 10:34.) He didn't love the people in the Bible more than He loves you. He isn't like other human beings who love some people, but don't love others.

Jesus doesn't want a member of your family to be sick the rest of his life. He wants to heal *you* and He wants to heal your family.

You must also get your belief settled that **the price for your healing has already been paid**. You don't have to wait for an evangelist to come to town to pray for you. You can have your healing now.

How To Approach God For Healing

Two things play an important role in how God manifests Himself and the amount of power He imparts to you to give you what you have asked for:

1. How you approach God.

2. What you say with your mouth.

Ask in Faith

The Holy Spirit will begin to move upon you when He finds favor in what you are doing. If you do exactly what the Bible says to do, then the Holy Spirit will encourage you because you are basing your actions on Scripture.

The way to get Jesus to manifest Himself is to ask for what you want in faith.

All through the New Testament, people boldly walked up to Jesus and said, "I want to be healed." There is no Scripture, from Matthew to Revelation, that says Jesus ever turned anyone away. He never said, "No. I'm not going to heal you." He touched anyone who asked Him for help and said, "Your faith has healed you." The deaf heard; the blind saw; the lame walked.

You have to show Jesus your faith; then He will heal you.

Know How To Receive His Healing Power

The same healing power that flowed through Jesus to open blind eyes and deaf ears is available for you today.

God's divine healing power is a substance exactly like His saving power. It flows automatically like a river, all through the air and everywhere in heaven. It is so strong that it can keep everything well.

After your spirit has been reborn by the Spirit of God, it is no longer a natural spirit. The Holy Ghost, who does all the work on the earth today, lives inside you. Whenever you believe the Bible, you enable God through the Holy Ghost to release His divine healing power (or whatever is needed) from heaven to your spirit here on earth. That healing power then flows from your spirit into your body and brings the healing or the miracle you need.

Several years ago, God put His healing power in my hands, and it has been there ever since. When it happened, I was speaking in Pennsylvania at a banquet in a Holiday Inn ballroom. The room was so full that people were standing around the walls.

A nice-looking fellow walked up to the front and said, "I'm a Full Gospel business-man here in town. I didn't know what was wrong with me until I heard you talk tonight. My ears have been stopped up for years and there is a knot in my belly about half as big as a football. I know now that there is a connection between the knot and my ears."

The Lord said to me, "Cast that deaf spirit out of him."

When an evil spirit has hold of a person, it won't let go very easily unless you command it to go with authority in Jesus' name. Then it has to go! It would inhabit a person for forty years if somebody didn't command it to leave.

I walked over to the man and said, "You foul deaf spirit, in Jesus' name, I command you to come out of him!"

The moment the Lord told me to cast out that deaf spirit, He put a great measure of His healing power in my hands. The man fell straight forward, face down on the floor. You would have thought all his teeth would have been knocked out, but they weren't.

Then he bounced and fell back down again. That impact could have broken his nose, but it didn't.

Again, he bounced up off the floor and fell back. This time he laid there real quiet for about sixty seconds. Then his mouth opened and a little squeaky sound like a mouse began to come out. It got louder, sounding like a big rat, and finally sounded like a screaming hyena.

In a little while the man shook his head and pushed himself up off the floor. He acted as if he had been hit in the head with a stick, but both ears had popped open and the knot in his stomach was gone!

The man had stepped up while I was still speaking. I hadn't given the invitation yet. Almost everybody at the banquet was from that town and they knew him. When the people—about 150 of them—saw that his ears had popped open and that the knot had disappeared, they jumped out of their seats and started running toward me, saying, "Pray for me!"

As I reached out and began to pray, it was as though the wind of God had come into my hands! People were lying all around on the floor, including denominational pastors. God baptized them in the Holy Ghost; and the moment they hit the floor, they started talking in tongues!

About five minutes later an old man walked up to me, stepping around the people who were lying crosswise and on top of each other on the floor. He told me what a blessing I was to him and said, "This is the first time in many years that I've seen this old-time power from heaven."

Do you know where you get that kind of power? From the Word of God.

Even though God may channel a great degree of healing power through you, you may not always feel it. Don't base whether or not you've been healed on your feelings.

Fred Price, pastor of Crenshaw Christian Center in Los Angeles, has a healing ministry in which about 98 percent of the people get healed. Why? Because he doesn't allow his congregation to operate according to their feelings.

After fifteen years in the ministry, Fred had about 350 people in his church. When he began to teach healing and faith from the Bible, his congregation grew in four years to 2200!

I have seen Fred pray for 100 people without anybody feeling anything. When he asks those who got healed to raise their hands, everybody except maybe one person holds up his hand. He then spends about ten minutes showing them from the Bible why they are already healed. His church draws people because everybody gets healed.

Fred teaches those 2200 people to believe God for everything. They open their Bibles and they tell the devil, and anybody else who asks, that they have what they are believing for—no matter how they feel or what they see.

Believe God's Word

Jesus said, *All things are possible to him that believeth* (Mark 9:23). God requires every person to believe the Bible and obey the Scriptures as they are written.

When God called me years ago, He said, "I want you to teach the Bible to the Church. I want you to teach them some things I've taught you. Everything I teach you, I'll give you a Scripture for."

Remember this: I don't have a "Norvel Hayes Gospel." You may think speaking in tongues and healing are strange because you have never been taught about them, but they are still in the Bible.

Maybe you've tried to make yourself believe in healing, but you can't. Maybe you've been taught another way for so long that it doesn't make any difference to you what the Bible says. But it does make a difference! *Faith cometh by hearing, and hearing by the word of God* (Rom. 10:17).

God doesn't go by what you have been taught. He goes according to what He has given you in the Bible. Read the Bible for yourself. Believe it on your own. God will bless you.

Believe and Confess

Hebrews 11:1 says, *Faith is the substance of things hoped for, the evidence of things not seen.* Regardless of how you feel, when you believe God, you have the substance: your faith, your believing.

Boldly confess what you are believing for, and God will work strongly for you. (2 Chron. 6:9.) He will give you everything you ask Him for. (John 15:7.)

Talk as though you've got it, and it will come. If you have to stop and think how to say it, then you don't really believe you've got it.

Nearly all Full Gospel Christians will say, "I believe that Jesus is going to heal me someday." But He is not obligated to do it as long as you talk like that. You are talking words of doubt.

With God "someday" never comes. Faith is right now. Stick your teeth into what you are believing for just like a tiger would stick his teeth into a piece of meat. Say boldly: "I've got it because God's Word says I have. It's mine now. I see it. I'm not *going* to get it; *I've got it right now!*"

James 1:6,7 says no one should think that he will receive anything from God if he wavers. To receive healing, you must have the "Abraham kind" of faith: be patient without doubting.

There was a time when my daughter had backslidden from God and was involved in dope and drugs. During the two years I prayed for her, she got even worse. After a healing service I had conducted in San Antonio, Texas, God told me my faith was wrong where my daughter was concerned. He said I was doubting.

In the meeting that night, people were healed all over the auditorium; but God said I had been doubting Him. How could that be? I found out that your faith can be strong in one area and weak in another.

God told me that the darkness over my daughter was too strong for her to come back to Him through her own faith; but He said that my faith could enable Him to visit her.

Attend A Church That Believes In Healing

If you want to be healed, you have to go to a church where the people believe in divine healing power. Your friends may be precious Christian people; but if their knowledge of

God's healing power isn't strong, you'd better not follow their advice about healing.

Southern Baptists have strong faith in salvation. If they ever memorize all the healing verses in the Bible and turn their faith loose on the sick people in town, everybody they pray for would probably get healed. But they don't have any faith in healing.

My family was Southern Baptist, and my mother loved Jesus. The Spirit of God would come on her with a glow of power that made her look like an angel. When that happened, she would shout without shame wherever she was—in a church or in a field.

Mother believed in God, but she didn't believe in divine healing. She died of cancer at 37. My brother, who was a football player in high school, died at 19 of Bright's disease, a disease of the kidneys.

There was no reason for them to die. Cancer is a lie, and God can give you new kidneys; but if you don't know that, you will suffer with your old infected kidneys (or whatever problem the devil puts on you).

If somebody had given my sweet Southern Baptist mother some of these healing verses, she would have believed them because she was open to God.

What To Do
For the Healing of Others

Be willing to do anything the Holy Spirit tells you to do. He may lead you into an unusual ministry that will get people saved and healed—people who otherwise would be lost and sick.

God will do anything with people who have His joy and power in them.

I heard a man and wife testify at a convention about an unusual ministry God had given them: cleaning filthy houses.

These are respectable, nice-looking people who live in a fine home; but every morning they go to skid row. The Lord shows them a filthy house that He wants them to clean. They go to the door and ask if they can scrub and clean at no charge—just to show their love. The people usually let them come in.

They never try to shove Jesus down the people's throats. While they take their time scrubbing and cleaning, they show their love and happily sing to the Lord.

Usually by noon the people are feeling convicted for the sins they have committed and begin to ask questions: "What are you people made out of? Why are you doing this? Because you love us? You don't even know us. How can you love us?

They answer, "Jesus loves you, and because Jesus is in us, He has given us His love for you." They win hundreds of souls to God through their cleaning ministry.

How To Pray For Healing

When you pray for healing, kneel down before Jesus and show God your faith. If you need a miracle in your life or healing for any kind of affliction in your body, kneel before Jesus and say, "Jesus, You are my healer."

Stick to the Scriptures when you pray. Don't try to dream up something new.

No matter what condition you may be in, God loves you just as much as He loved the people in the Bible. When you pay the same price as those people did, you will get the same results.

Kneel down before God. Cry out for Him to have mercy on you, and God Almighty will heal you. Why? Because the Bible says He will.

I Pray This For You...

In the name of the Lord Jesus Christ, I pray for you now.

I rise up against the devil and his power over you. In Jesus' name, I command Satan to let you go free! I command the foul devils that have wrecked your life and bound you up with sickness and disease to let you go free!

Jesus said you can't come to Him unless the Spirit draws you, so I pray now that the Holy Spirit will melt your heart and make you sensitive to God.

I command all darkness to flee from you. I pray that the light of God will shine on you and the Spirit of the Living God will wash you white as snow. I accept it in faith as done now, in Jesus' name.

Thank You, Jesus, that You hear my prayer.

Know That He Hears Your Prayers

The Spirit of God once showed me how you can know when your prayer has been answered. After you have prayed long enough, the Holy Ghost will begin to laugh inside you. Joy will start bubbling up supernaturally.

God loves you and He wants you to know it! Approach Him in reverence and faith, and He will lead you!

Healing Scriptures

My son, attend to my words; incline thine ear unto my sayings. Let them not depart from thine eyes; keep them in the midst of thine heart. For they are life unto those that find them, and health to all their flesh.

Proverbs 4:20-22

Behold, I will bring health and cure, and I will heal them, and will reveal unto them the abundance of peace and truth.

Jeremiah 33:6

...Thus saith the Lord, the God of David thy father, I have heard thy prayer, I have seen thy tears: behold, I will heal thee.

2 Kings 20:5

Be not wise in thine own eyes: fear the Lord, and depart from evil. It will be health (medicine) *to thy navel, and marrow* (refreshment) *to thy bones.*

Proverbs 3:7,8

And ye shall serve the Lord your god, and he shall bless thy bread, and thy water; and I will take sickness from the midst of thee.

Exodus 23:25

Now when the sun was setting, all they that had any sick with divers diseases brought them unto him; and he laid hands on every one of them, and healed them.

Luke 4:40

And Jesus went forth, and saw a great multitude, and was moved with compassion toward them, and he healed their sick.

Matthew 14:14

...they brought unto him many that were possessed with devils: and he cast out the spirits with his word, and healed all that were sick.

Matthew 8:16

...they brought unto him all sick people that were taken with divers diseases and torments...and he healed them.

Matthew 4:24

And the prayer of faith shall save the sick, and the Lord shall raise him up.

James 5:15

Who his own self bare our sins in his own body on the tree, that we, being dead to sins, should live unto righteousness: by whose stripes ye were healed.

1 Peter 2:24

He was wounded for our transgressions, he was bruised for our iniquities: the chastisement of our peace was upon him; and with his stripes we are healed.

Isaiah 53:5

And when I passed by thee, and saw thee polluted in thine own blood, I said unto thee when thou wast in thy blood, Live: yea, I said unto thee when thou wast in thy blood, Live.

Ezekiel 16:6

...I will put none of these diseases upon thee...for I am the Lord that healeth thee.

Exodus 15:26

Bless the Lord, O my soul, and forget not all his benefits: Who forgiveth all thine iniquities; who healeth all thy diseases.

Psalm 103:2,3

For I will restore health unto thee, and I will heal thee of thy wounds, saith the Lord.

Jeremiah 30:17

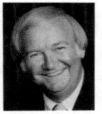

Norvel Hayes

Norvel Hayes is a successful businessman, internationally renowned Bible teacher, and founder of several Christian ministries in the U.S. and abroad.

Brother Hayes founded *New Life Bible College,* located in Cleveland, Tennessee, in 1977. *New Life Bible Church* grew out of the Bible school's chapel services. The Bible School offers a two-year diploma and off-campus correspondence courses. Among it's many other out-reaches, the church ministers God's Word and hot meals daily to the poor through the *New Life Soup Kitchen.*

Brother Hayes is also the founder and president of *New Life Maternity Home,* a ministry dedicated to the spiritual, physical and financial need of young girls during pregnancy; *Campus Challenge,* and evangelistic outreach that distributes Christian literature on college campuses across America; *Street Reach,* a ministry dedicated to runaway teens located in Daytona Beach, Florida; and *Children's Home,* an orphanage home and education center located in India.

Known internationally for his dynamic exposition of the Word of God, Brother Hayes spends most of his time teaching and ministering God's deliverance and healing power in churches, college classrooms, conventions and seminars around the world.

For a complete list of tapes and books by Norvel Hayes, write:

Norvel Hayes • P. O. Box 1379 • Cleveland, TN 37311

Books by Norvel Hayes

Don't Let the Devil Steal Your Destiny

How to Live and Not Die

Worship

The Blessing of Obedience

The Chosen Fast

Confession Brings Possession

How To Get Your Prayers Answered

Let Not Your Heart Be Troubled

Misguided Faith

The Number One Way To Fight the Devil

What To Do for Healing

Available from your local bookstore.
HARRISON HOUSE
P.O. Box 35035
Tulsa, OK 74153

The Harrison House Vision

Proclaiming the truth and the power
Of the Gospel of Jesus Christ
With excellence;
Challenging Christians to
Live victoriously,
Grow spiritually,
Know God intimately.